The Consumer Guide To
FINDING FREE OR LOW COST
HEALTHCARE IN ARKANSAS

CONSUMER GUIDE TO FINDING FREE OR LOW COST HEALTHCARE IN ARKANSAS

Law Offices of Lisa Douglas, Inc.
2300 Main
North Little Rock, AR 72114
501-798-0004
www.LisaGDouglas.com

TABLE OF CONTENTS:

Foreword
WHY THIS BOOK?

I wrote this book to assist Social Security Applicants in finding medical treatment. In order to prove your disability, a claimant must have the adequate medical documentation to prove their claim. Without this necessary documentation, the claimant is not able to prove their claim. Many of the claimants do not have healthcare coverage and lack the funds to pay for any healthcare.

Because this healthcare and the documentation that results is so vital to your claim it is essential to receive this healthcare. If you are like most, this is the first time you have resorted to the system that you paid into and now lack the funds to prove up your case, because you cannot afford the healthcare. That is why I wrote this book, to equip you with the resources to pursue the healthcare and medical documentation to prove up your case.

I wrote this book for you. Hopefully you will find it a valuable tool that will give you some valuable information to consider while you are seeking healthcare.

This book is too limited to explore every issue or address each possible question you may have.

Further, this book is not intended to give legal advice and nothing in this book is legal advice. Obtaining this book from me does not create an attorney client- relationship between us. I do not sign up everyone who calls my office that has a social security claim.

This book lists both federally funded health care centers and free to low cost clinics.

Federally-funded health centers care for

you, even if you have no health
insurance. You pay what you can afford,
based on your income.

These federally funded health centers
provide primary medical and dental care
to people of all ages, whether or not they
have health insurance.

The Health Resources and Services
Administration (HRSA) is an agency
within the U.S. Department of Health
and Human Services. Millions of
Americans receive affordable health
care through HRSA programs.

These federally funded health Centers
can be found at http://www.hrsa.gov
and are designated by *astericks in this
book.

Additional Free Clinics or Low Cost
Clinics can be found at:
http://freeclinicdirectory.org/arkansas_
care.html
These clinics are designated by + in this

book.
Another online source to locate free clinics can be found at:
http://www.freemedicalsearch.org/sta/arkansas
or
www.freemedicalcamps.com **Or** http://www.nafcclinics.org **(National Association of Free and Charitable Clinics)**

For more information on free clinics or to find out how you can help at a free clinic, go to http://www.freeclinics.us

County: Arkansas County, AR

ELMER & GLADYS FERGUSON RURAL
HEALTH CLINIC
1641 S. Whitehead Dr.
De Witt AR 72042
870-946-3637

County: Ashley County, AR

ASHLEY HEALTH SERVICES - Ashley County
Medical Center
1003 Fred Lagrone Dr.
Crossett AR 71635
870-364-8062

*MAINLINE HEALTH SYSTEM, INC.
233 N Main St
Portland, AR 71663-9230
Telephone Number: 870-737-2221
Appointment Number: 870-737-2737 x21

MAINLINE HEALTH SYSTEMS - Wilmot
203 McComb St.
Wilmot AR 71676
Website: http://www.mainlinehealth.net
870-473-2274

+FOUNTAIN HILL MAINLINE
127 N. Hickory St.
Fountain Hill, AR 71642
Number: 870-853-9993

*WILMOT CLINIC
203 McCombs
Wilmot, AR 71676-8800
Telephone Number: 870-473-2274
Appointment Number: 870-737-2737 x21

County: Baxter County, AR

MOUNTAIN HOME CHRISTIAN CLINIC
421 W. Wade St.
Mountain Home AR 72653
website: http://www.mountainhomechristianclinic.org
870-425-5010

STONE COUNTY PRIMARY CARE CLINIC
2202 East Main Street
Mountain View AR 72560

Website: http://www.whiteriverhealthsystem.com
Telephone:870-269-6495

County: Benton County, AR

*COMMUNITY CLINIC ROGERS MEDICAL
1233 W Poplar St
Rogers, AR 72756-4245
Website: www.communityclinicnwa.org
Telephone Number: 479-636-9235
Appointment Number: 479-751-7417 x6069

*COMMUNITY CLINIC ROGERS/DENTAL
3710 Southern Hills Blvd
Rogers, AR 72758-8041
Website: www.communityclinicnwa.org
Telephone Number: 479-936-8600
Appointment Number: 479-751-7417 x6069

COMMUNITY CLINIC AT ST. FRANCIS HOUSE
614 E. Emma 300
Springdale AR 72764
855-438-2280

*COMMUNITY CLINIC SILOAM SPRINGS
MEDICAL
500 S Mount Olive St Ste 200
Siloam Springs, AR 72761-3602
Website: www.communityclinicnwa.org
Telephone Number: 479-524-9550

DECATUR MEDI CLINIC
346 N. Main
Decatur AR 72722
479-752-3233

MERCY CLINIC PRIMARY CARE - CENTERTON
805 W. Centerton Boulevard
Centerton AR 72719
479-795-1301

CENMERCY CLINIC FAMILY MEDICINE - LOWELL
325 S. 6th
Lowell AR 72745
479-770-0700

MERCY CLINIC GASTROENTEROLOGY -
MONROE AVENUE
116 W. Monroe Avenue
Lowell AR 72745
479-770-8090

MERCY CLINIC FAMILY MEDICINE - W. ELM
1110 W. Elm
Rogers AR 72756
479-878-1060

MERCY CLINIC FAMILY MEDICINE AND
OBSTERICS - PHYSICIAN PLAZA
2708 Rife Medical Lane
Rogers AR 72758

479-338-5555

SAMARITAN HOUSE COMMUNITY CENTER
1211 W. Hudson Road
Rogers AR 72756

479-636-4198

County: Boone County, AR

CLAUDE PARRISH COMMUNITY HEALTH CLINIC
131 Highway 14 E.
Lead Hill AR 72644
Telephone Number: 870-436-5271

+THE MEDICAL CLINIC MISSION OF
HARRISON ARKANSAS
1400 South Pine Street
Harrison, AR 72601
Telephone Number: 870-365-0341

County: Calhoun County, AR

*CABUN RURAL HEALTH SERVICES, INC.
402 N Lee St
Hampton, AR 71744-8937

Website: cabun.org
Telephone Number: 870-798-4299
Appointment Number: 870-798-4064

County: Carroll County, AR

*BOSTON MOUNTAIN RURAL HEALTH
CENTER, INC.
1103 E Main St
Green Forest, AR 72638-2810
Website: bmrhc.org
Appointment Number: 870-448-3796

ECHO Free Clinic (Eureka Christian Health Outreach)
4004 East Van Buren
Eureka Springs AR 72632
479-253-5547

MERCY CLINIC ORTHOPEDICS - GREEN FOREST
100 Medical Circle
Green Forest AR 72638
877-400-0770

MERCY CLINIC FAMILY MEDICINE - HOLIDAY
ISLAND
1 Park Drive Unit 203
Holiday Island AR 72631
479-363-9174

County: Chicot County, AR

*DERMOTT MEDICAL AND DENTAL CLINIC
300 S School St
Dermott, AR 71638-2127
Telephone Number: 870-538-3355
Appointment Number: 870-538-3355 x26

*EUDORA CLINIC
579 E Beouff St
Eudora, AR 71640-3090
Telephone Number: 870-355-2512
Appointment Number: 870-737-2737 x21

LAKE VILLAGE CLINIC
2918 Louis Sessions St.
Lake Village AR 71653
Telephone Number: 870-265-5348

MAINLINE HEALTH SYSTEMS - DERMOTT
300 South School Street
Dermott AR 71638
Website: http://www.mainlinehealth.net
870-538-3355

MAINLINE HEALTH SYSTEMS - EUDORA
579 East Beouff St.
Eudora AR 71640
870-355-2512

County: Clark County, AR

*AMITY COMMUNITY HEALTH CENTER
329 N Hill St
Amity, AR 71921-9635
Website: cabun.org
Telephone Number: 870-342-5606
Appointment Number: 870-798-4064

County: Clay County, AR
*CORNING AREA HEALTHCARE, INC.
1300 Creason Rd
Corning, AR 72422-1716
Telephone Number: 870-857-3399
Appointment Number: 870-857-3399 x222

County: Cleburne County, AR
*ARcare - 85
1511 Highway 25B
Heber Springs, AR 72543-1701
Website: www.arcare.net
Telephone Number: 501-362-9426
Appointment Number: 870-347-2534

+HEBER SPRINGS FAMILY HEALTH
CENTER
1716 West Searcy
Heber Springs, AR 72543
Telephone Number: 501-362-7595

+CHRISTIAN HEALTH CENTER
501 West Main
Heber Springs, AR 72543
Telephone Number: 501-362-2252

DRASCO MEDICAL CLINIC
60 Greers Ferry Road
Drasco AR 72530
870-668-3200

HEBER SPRINGS MEDICAL CLINIC (ARCARE)
1511 Highway 25B A
Heber Springs AR 72543
501-362-9426

County: Cleveland County, AR

RISON CLINIC
505 Sycamore
Rison AR 71665
Telephone Number: 870-325-6255

County: Craighead County, AR

LAKE CITY MEDICAL CLINIC (ARCARE)
1009 Highway 18
Lake City AR 72437
Telephone Number: 870-237-9928

*JONESBORO FAMILY HC - NORTH
1530 N Church St
Jonesboro, AR 72401-1515
Website: www.wrrhc-ar.org
Telephone Number: 870-802-3586
Appointment Number: 870-347-2534

*JONESBORO FAMILY HEALTH CENTER -
SOUTH
2816 Fox Meadow Ln
Jonesboro, AR 72404-9346
Website: www.wrrhc-ar.org
Telephone Number: 870-336-1675
Appointment Number: 870-347-2534

JONESBORO CHURCH HEALTH CENTER
200 W. Matthews Ave. PO Box 924
Jonesboro AR 72401
Telephone Number: 870-972-4777

*LAKE CITY HEALTH CENTER

1009 Highway 18

Lake City, AR 72437-9622

Website: www.wrrhc-ar.org

Telephone Number: 870-237-3399

Appointment Number: 870-347-2534

Appointment Number: 870-237-9928

County: Crawford County, AR

MERCY CLINIC FAMILY MEDICINE - VAN BUREN
2800 Fayetteville Road
Van Buren AR 72956

Website: http://www.mercy.net
479-314-4000

*MOUNTAINBURG FAMILY CLINIC

4 Highway 71 N

Mountainburg, AR 72946

Website: www.rvpcs.org/

Telephone Number: 479-369-2091

Appointment Number: 479-635-0091 x240

*MULBERRY FAMILY CLINIC

437 N Main St

Mulberry, AR 72947-8574

Website: http://www.rvpcs.org

Telephone Number: 479-997-1484

Appointment Number: 479-635-0091 x240

County: Crittenden County,

ARKANSAS DELTA AIDS CARE CENTER - EAFHC
210 North 6th Street
West Memphis AR 72301

Website: http://www.eafhc.org
870-735-3291

*EAST ARKANSAS FAMILY HEALTH CENTER, INC.
215 E Bond Ave
West Memphis, AR 72301-3550
Website: eafhc.org
Telephone Number: 870-735-3842
Appointment Number: 870-732-6520

County: Cross County, AR

CHERRY VALLEY MEDICAL CLINIC (ARCARE)
2624 Hwy 42
Cherry Valley AR 72324
855-497-7271

*PARKIN MEDICAL CLINIC & PHARMACY-ARCARE

1740 Church St

Parkin, AR 72373

Website: www.wrrhc-ar.org

Telephone Number: 870-755-2234

Appointment Number: 870-347-2534

*WYNNE HEALTH CENTER

611 Julia Ave E

Wynne, AR 72396-3506

Website: www.wrrhc-ar.org

Telephone Number: 870-238-0377

County: Desha County, AR

DE PAUL HEALTH CENTER OF DUMAS
145 W. Waterman St.
Dumas AR 71639
870-382-4878

Delta Health Services
811 Highway 65 S.
Dumas AR 71639
870-382-8261

UAMS
803 Highway 65 South
Dumas, AR 71639
Telephone Number: 870-382-2091

County: Drew County, AR

*MONTICELLO COMMUNITY HEALTH
CENTER
766 H L Ross Dr
Monticello, AR 71655-5706
Website: http://www.mainlinehealth.net

(870) 367-MAIN(6246)

County: Faulkner County, AR

BANISTER LIEBLONG CLINIC
2425 Dave Ward Dr. 410
Conway AR 72034
501-329-3824

CONWAY INTERFAITH CLINIC
830 North Creek
Conway AR 72032
501-932-0559

CONWAY MEDICAL CLINIC
1500 Museum Rd. Ste. 104
Conway AR 72032
501-932-9010

PINE STREET FREE CLINIC
1114 Ingram Street
Conway AR 72032
501-932-0989

County: Franklin County, AR

MERCY CLINIC FAMILY MEDICINE - OZARK
201 S. 7th Street
Ozark AR 72949
479-667-1590

County: Fulton County, AR

MAMMOTH SPRING MEDICAL CLINIC -
OZARKS MEDICAL CENTER
260 S. Main St.
Mammoth Spring AR 72554
870-625-3228

FAMILY HEALTH CARE
350 S. Main St. Suite 4
Mammoth Spring AR 72554
870-625-3111

SALEM 1ST CARE - OZARKS MEDICAL CENTER
172 Highway 62 E. 1
Salem AR 72576
870-895-1911

County: Garland County, AR

CHARITABLE CHRISTIAN MEDICAL CLINIC
133 Arbor St.
Hot Springs AR 71901
501-623-8850

MERCY CLINIC CARDIOLOGY - HEART CENTER
200 Heart Center Lane
Hot Springs AR 71913
501-624-6641

MERCY CLINIC CARDIOLOGY - HOT
SPRINGS VILLAGE
4419 N. Highway 7
Hot Springs AR 71909
501-624-6641

MERCY CLINIC EAR, NOSE AND THROAT -
MAIN CAMPUS
One Mercy Lane Stge 106
Hot Springs AR 71913

501-609-2368

MERCY CLINIC FAMILY INTERNAL MEDICINE
AND PEDIATRICS- 70 West
1707 Airport Road
Hot Springs AR 71913
501-767-6200

MERCY CLINIC FAMILY MEDICINE -
MCGOWAN COURT
100 McGowan Court
Hot Springs AR 71913
501-627-1800

MERCY CLINIC FAMILY PRACTICE - MAIN CAMPUS
One Mercy Lane Ste 506
Hot Springs AR 71913
501-622-6500

MERCY CLINIC INTERNAL MEDICINE - HOT
SPRINGS VILLAGE
4419 N. Highway 7
Hot Springs AR 71909
501-922-2217

MERCY CLINIC INTERNAL MEDICINE -
SOUTH CAMPUS

1662 Higdon Ferry Road
Hot Springs AR 71913
501-623-2781

MERCY CLINIC ONCOLOGY - HOT SPRINGS
1455 Higdon Ferry Road
Hot Springs AR 71913
501-623-2731

MERCY CLINIC PEDIATRICS - MCAULEY COURT
225 McAuley Court
Hot Springs AR 71913
501-321-2546

MERCY CLINIC RHEUMATOLOGY -
MCGOWAN COURT
100 McGowan Court
Hot Springs AR 71913
501-627-1800

MERCY CONVENIENT CARE - CENTRAL AVENUE
3604 Central Avenue
Hot Springs AR 71913
501-525-9675

MERCY GERIATRIC PSYCHIATRIC SERVICES - HOT SPRINGS
300 Werner Street
Hot Springs AR 71903
501-622-1291

MERCY INTENSIVE OUTPATIENT PSYCHIATRIC SERVICES - SURGERY CENTER
1636 Higdon Ferry Road
Hot Springs AR 71913
501-520-3771

MERCY MCAULE CLINIC - HOLLYWOOD AVENUE
104 Hollywood Avenue
Hot Springs AR 71901
501-321-2055

MERCY CONVENIENT CARE - SENIOR CENTER
5010 Highway 7 North
Hot Springs Village AR 71909
501-984-6780

MERCY SPECIALTY SERVICES - DESOTO
903 DeSoto Boulevard
Hot Springs Village AR 71909
501-922-2680

County: Greene County, AR

MISSION OUTREACH OF NORTHEAST ARKANSAS - CHARITABLE MEDICAL CLINIC
#1 Medical Drive
Paragould AR 72450
Website:
http://missionoutreachnea.com/services/

870-236-8080

PARAGOULD DOCTORS CLINIC
1 Medical Dr. Ste 100
Paragould AR 72450
870-239-8503

County: Hempstead County, AR

*HOPE MIGRANT HEALTH CENTER
205 Smith Rd
Hope, AR 71801-8801
Website: cabun.org
Telephone Number: 870-777-8420
Appointment Number: 870-798-4064

County: Hot Sprigs County, AR

MERCY CLINIC FAMILY MEDICINE - MALVERN
1424 Tanner Street

Malvern AR 72104
501-332-8612

County: Howard County, AR

CHRISTIAN HEALTH CENTER OF HOWARD COUNTY
121 West Sypert St
Nashville AR 71852
Website: http://www.nafcclinics.org
870-845-2871

County: Independence County, AR

*INDEPENDENCE FAMILY HEALTH
1183 Batesville Blvd
Batesville, AR 72501-8925
Website: www.wrrhc-ar.org
Telephone Number: 870-347-2534
Appointment Number: 870-347-2534

*INDEPENDENCE FAMILY HEALTH CENTER
1175 Vine St BPHC
Batesville, AR 72501-3526
Website: www.wrrhc-ar.org
Telephone Number: 870-251-9933
Appointment Number: 870-347-2534

NEWARK MEDICAL CLINIC
501 Vine St.
Newark AR 72562
Website: http://www.whiteriverhealthsystem.com
870-799-3299

PLEASANT PLAINS MEDICAL CLINIC
6200 Batesville Blvd.
Pleasant Plains AR 72568
501-345-2182

County: Izard County, AR

MELBOURNE MEDICAL CLINIC
1526 E. Main St.
Melbourne AR 72556
870-368-4344

County: Jackson County, AR

CHRISTIAN COMMUNITY CLINIC OF
JACKSON COUNTY
1420 McLain St
Newport AR 72112
870-523-7505

NEWPORT DIAGNOSTIC MED. CLINIC
2200 Malcolm Ave Ste. B

Newport AR 72112
870-512-2500

*NEWPORT MEDICAL CLINIC - ARCARE
1507 N Pecan St
Newport, AR 72112-2867
Website: www.arcare.net
Telephone Number: 870-523-2944
Appointment Number: 870-347-2534

*SWIFTON MEDICAL CLINIC
300 E Main St
Swifton, AR 72471
Website: www.wrrhc-ar.org
Telephone Number: 870-485-2234
Appointment Number: 870-347-2534

County: Jefferson County, AR

*ALTHEIMER CLINIC
309 S Edline
Altheimer, AR 72004-8559
Telephone Number: 870-766-8411
Appointment Number: 870-543-2315

*REDFIELD CLINIC
113 W River Rd
Redfield, AR 72132-9253
Telephone Number: 501-397-2261
Appointment Number: 870-543-2315

+JEFFERSON COMPREHENSIVE CARE SYS-
TEM
1101 Tennessee Street
Pine Bluff, AR 71601
Telephone Number: 870-543-2309
Telephone Number: 870-543-2380

PINE BLUFF MEDICAL & DENTAL CENTER - JCCSI
1101 Tennessee St
Pine Bluff AR 71613
website: http://www.jccsi.org
870-543-2380

County: Lafayette County, AR

*+LEWISVILLE FAMILY PRACTICE CTR.
1117 Chestnut St
Lewisville, AR 71845
Website: cabun.org
Telephone Number: 870-921-5781
Appointment Number: 870-798-4064

County: Lawrence County, AR

*COMMUNITY HEALTHCARE CENTER
3219 Highway 67B
Walnut Ridge, AR 72476-8567
Telephone Number: 870-886-5507
Appointment Number: 870-857-3399

HOXIE MEDICAL CLINIC - LAWRENCE HEALTH
505 S.E. Lindsey St.
Hoxie AR 72433
870-886-4711

County: Lee County, AR

LAWRENCE HEALTH/RURAL HEALTH CLINIC
1309 W. Main St.
Walnut Ridge AR 72476
870-886-3211

*+LEE COUNTY COOPERATIVE CLINIC
530 Atkins Blvd
Marianna, AR 72360-2113
Telephone Number: 870-295-5225
Appointment Number: 870-295-5225

STRAWBERRY MEDICAL CLINIC
58 River Drive
Strawberry AR 72469
870-528-4081

County: Lincoln County, AR

ST ELIZABETH HEALTH CENTER
407 S Gould Ave
Gould AR 71643

870-263-4317

County: Logan County, AR

*+RIVER VALLEY PRIMARY CARE SERVICES
INC.
9755 W State Highway 22
Ratcliff, AR 72951-9000
Website: www.rvpcs.org
Telephone Number: 479-635-5300 x240
Appointment Number: 479-635-0091

County: Lonoke County, AR

*ARCARE - 93
614 N Grant St BPHC
Cabot, AR 72023-2656
Website: www..arcare.net
Telephone Number: 870-347-2534
Appointment Number: 870-347-2534

CABOT MEDICAL CLINIC - ARCARE
614 North Grant Street
Cabot AR 72023
501-941-3522

*+CARLISLE MEDICAL CLINIC-ARCARE
821 East Park St Hwy 70

Carlisle, AR 72024
Website: www.wrrhc-ar.org
Telephone Number: 870-552-7303
Appointment Number: 870-347-2534

*ENGLAND HEALTH CENTER-ARCARE
227 Pine Bluff Hwy
England, AR 72046-2234
Website: www.arcare.net
Telephone Number: 501-842-3131
Lonoke County Christian Clinic
502 Richie Rd. PO Box 1102
Cabot AR 72023
501-605-5600

County: Madison County, AR

***+BOSTON MOUNTAIN RURAL HEALTH
CENTER, INC.**
934 N Gaskill St
Huntsville, AR 72740-8903
Website: www.bmrhc.org
Telephone Number: 479-738-5500
Appointment Number: 870-448-3796

County: Marion County, AR

**BOSTON MOUNTAIN RURAL HEALTH
CENTER, INC. YELLVILLE**
358 East Valley Street

Yellville AR 72687
870-449-7000

County: Mississippi County, AR

CULLOM RURAL HEALTH CLINIC
700 W. Keiser Ave.
Osceola AR 72370
870-563-6512

*HEALTHY PARTNERS
4102 Memorial Dr
Blytheville, AR 72315-5771
Website: eafhc.org
Telephone Number: 870-532-6001
Appointment Number: 870-732-6520

WAGNER MEDICAL CLINIC
434 W. St Hwy 18 Bypass
Manila AR 72442
870-561-3300

County: Monroe County, AR

*BRINKLEY HEALTH CENTER & PHARMACY
615 N Main St
Brinkley, AR 72021-2507
Website: www.wrrhc-ar.org
Telephone Number: 870-734-1150

Appointment Number: 870-347-2534

*+MID-DELTA HEALTH SYSTEMS, INC.
401 Midland St
Clarendon, AR 72029-2727
Telephone Number: 870-747-3381
Appointment Number: 870-747-3381 x226

+HOLLY GROVE HEALTH CENTER
106 South Smith Street
Holly Grove, AR 72069
Telephone Number: 870-462-3393

County: Montgomery County, AR

*MONTGOMERY COUNTY COMMUNITY
CLINIC
534 Luzerne St
Mount Ida, AR 71957-9449
Website: www.healthy-connections.org
Telephone Number: 870-867-4244 x118
Appointment Number: 479-394-2332 x500

County: Newton County, AR

*BOSTON MOUNTAIN RURAL HEALTH CTR
Hc 31 Box 310
Deer, AR 72628-9616
Website: www.bmrhc.org
Telephone Number: 870-428-5391

Appointment Number: 870-448-3796

County: Ouachita County, AR

*+BEARDEN HEALTH CENTER
2nd & School Street
Bearden, AR 71720
Website: cabun.org
Telephone Number: 870-687-3637
Appointment Number: 870-798-4064

CHRISTIAN HEALTH CENTER
1115 Fairview
Camden AR 71701
870-231-1111

STEPHENS COMMUNITY CLINIC
113 W. Ruby St.
Stephens AR 71764
870-786-9114

County: Phillips County, AR

HELENA FAMILY HEALTH CENTER - EAFHC
513 Porter Street
Helena AR 72342
870-817-0122

*LAKEVIEW AREA CLINIC
14264 Highway 44

Helena, AR 72342-9070
Telephone Number: 870-827-3201
Appointment Number: 870-295-5225

PHILLIPS COUNTY HEALTH CENTER
110 Shirley Hicks Lane
West Helena AR 72390
870-572-9028

THE PILLOW CLINIC
1008 Main St.
Marvell AR 72366
870-829-2521

County: Pike County, AR

MERCY CLINIC FAMILY MEDICINE - GLENWOOD
234 Broadway
Glenwood AR 71943
870-356-4821

MERCY CLINIC FAMILY MEDICINE - MURFREESBORO
319 E.13th Street
Murfreesboro AR 71958
Website: http://www.mercy.net
Telephone: 870-285-3118

County: Poinsett County, AR

*+EAST ARKANSAS FAMILY HEALTH CTR
102 W Broad St
Lepanto, AR 72354-2200
Website: eafhc.org
Telephone Number: 870-475-2977
Appointment Number: 870-732-6520

LEPANTO FAMILY HEALTH CENTER - EAFHC
102 West Broad Street
Lepanto AR 72354
Telephone Number: 870-475-2977

*TRUMAN FAMILY HEALTH CENTER
417 W Main St
Trumann, AR 72472-3116
website: http://www.eafhc.org
Telephone Number: 870-483-1025

County: Polk County, AR

***WESTERN ARKANSAS TOTAL
COMMUNITY HEALTH CENTER (WATCH)**
1201 Mena St
Mena, AR 71953-4280
Website: www.healthy-connections.org
Telephone Number: 479-437-3449

Appointment Number: 394-394-2332 x500

+HEALTHY CONNECTIONS
Healthy Connections - Mena
136 Health Park Dr PO Box 1848
Mena AR 71953
Website: http://www.healthy-connections.org
Telephone Number: 479-437-3449

NINTH STREET MINISTRY FREE CLINIC
811 Port Arthur Ave.
Mena AR 71953
Website: http://handtohandfoundation.com
Telephone Number: 479-394-2541

County: Prairie County, AR

DES ARC MEDICAL CLINIC (ARCARE)
405 Highway 11 N
Des Arc AR 72040
870-256-3009

*+DES ARC DENTAL CLINIC
405 Highway 11 N
Des Arc, AR 72040-3140
Website: www.wrrhc-ar.org
Telephone Number: 870-256-3009
Appointment Number: 870-347-2534

*+DES ARC HEALTH CENTER
405 Highway 11 N
Des Arc, AR 72040-3140
Website: www.wrrhc-ar.org
Telephone Number: 870-256-4178
Appointment Number: 870-347-2534

*+HAZEN MEDICAL CLINIC
100 E Front St
Hazen, AR 72064
Website: www.wrrhc-ar.org
Telephone Number: 870-255-3696
Appointment Number: 870-347-2534

MID DELTA HEALTH CENTER
693 Market St.
De Valls Bluff AR 72041
870-998-2571

County: Pulaski County, AR

*COLLEGE STATION CLINIC
4206 Frazier Pike
College Station, AR
Telephone Number: 501-490-2440
Appointment Number: 870-543-2315

ESPERANZA HOPE CLINIC
6111 W 83rd St

Little Rock AR 72209
Telephone Number: 501-562-1114

GARDNER MEMORIAL CLINIC
1723 Schaer
North Little Rock AR 72114
website: http://www.gardnermemorialumc.org
501-552-3241

GLENVIEW COMMUNITY CLINIC
4800 East 19th St
North Little Rock AR 72117
website: https://www.stvincenthealth.com
501-552-3241

*HOMELESS OPEN HANDS
1225 Dr Martin Luther King Dr
Little Rock, AR 72202-4743
Telephone Number: 501-244-2121
Appointment Number: 870-543-2315

*LITTLE ROCK CHC
1522 W 10th St
Little Rock, AR 72202-3526
Telephone Number: 501-376-1285
Appointment Number: 870-543-2315

+COMMUNITY HEALTH CENTERS OF
ARKANSAS

420 West 4th Street, Suite A
North Little Rock, AR 72114
Telephone Number: 501-374-8225

+CAMP ALDERSGATE
2000 Aldersgate Rd.
Little Rock, AR 72205
Telephone Number: 501-664-0340 ext. 356

+HARMONY HEALTH CLINIC
201 East Roosevelt
Little Rock, AR 72206
Telephone Number: 501-375-4400

RIVER CITY CLINIC
1021 East Washington Ave
North Little Rock AR 72113
website: http://www.rivercityministry.org/
501-376-6694

ST. FRANCIS HOUSE CLINIC
2701 South Elm St.
Little Rock AR 72204
Telephone Number: 501-552-3241

SHEPHERD'S HOPE NEIGHBORHOOD
HEALTH CENTER
2404 S. Tyler St.
Little Rock AR 72204

Telephone Number: 501-614-9523

County: Randolph County, AR

*+POCAHONTAS FAMILY MEDICAL CENTER
141 Betty Dr
Pocahontas, AR 72455-3602
Telephone Number: 870-892-9949
Appointment Number: 870-857-3399

County: Scott County, AR

MERCY CLINIC FAMILY MEDICINE - WALDRON
1341 W. 6th St.
Waldron AR 72958
479-637-4135

County: St. Francis County, AR

*+HUGHES CLINIC
503 S Broadway St
Hughes, AR 72348-9701
Telephone Number: 870-339-4181
Appointment Number: 870-295-5225

County: Searcy County, AR

*+BOSTON MOUNTAIN RURAL HEALTH
CENTER
2263 Highway 65 N

Marshall, AR 72650
Website: www.bmrhc.org
Telephone Number: 870-448-5733
Appointment Number: 870-448-3796

BOSTON MOUNTAIN RURAL HEALTH
CENTER, INC. - WELLNESS CENTER
400 Highway 27 South
Marshall AR 72650
870-448-5733

County: Sebastian County, AR

COMMUNITY DENTAL CLINIC
109 N. 17th St
Fort Smith AR 72901
479-782-6021

HEMBREE CANCER CENTER
7301 Rogers Avenue
Fort Smith AR 72903
479-314-7545

MERCY CLINIC CARDIOLOGY - PHOENIX AVENUE
6101 Phoenix Avenue
Fort Smith AR 72903
479-452-1188

MERCY CLINIC CARDIOLOGY - ROGERS AVENUE
7001 Rogers Avenue Ste 401A
Fort Smith AR 72903
479-314-4650

MERCY CLINIC HYPERBARICS AND WOUND CARE - FORT SMITH
7301 Rogers Avenue
Fort Smith AR 72903
479-314-2804

MERCY CLINIC INTERNAL MEDICINE AND PEDIATRICS - MASSARD ROAD
4107 Massard Road
Fort Smith AR 72903
479-314-4940

MERCY CLINIC OB/GYN - 70TH STREET
3224 S. 70th Street
Fort Smith AR 72903
479-785-2229

MERCY CLINIC ONCOLOGY - FORT SMITH
7001 Rogers Avenue
Fort Smith AR 72903
479-314-7490

MERCY CLINIC ORTHOPEDICS -
NEUROSURGERY- PODIATRY -
OUTPATIENT SURGERY CENTER RIVER VALLEY
3501 W. E Knight Drive
Fort Smith AR 72903
479-709-6700

MERCY CLINIC ORTHOPEDICS - RIVER VALLEY
3501 W. E Knight Drive
Fort Smith AR 72903
479-709-6700

MERCY CLINIC PEDIATRICS - FORT SMITH
7303 Rogers Avenue Ste 200
Fort Smith AR 72903
479-314-4810

MERCY CLINIC PRIMARY CARE - DALLAS STREET
7800 Dallas St.
Fort Smith AR 72903
479-221-9922

MERCY CLINIC PULMONOLOGY - FORT SMITH
7001 Rogers Avenue
Fort Smith AR 72903
479-314-4620

MERCY URGENT CARE - RIVER VALLEY
3500 W.E. Knight Drive
Fort Smith AR 72903
479-709-8686

MERCY FAMILY MEDICINE - MANSFIELD
103 Huntington Ave
Mansfield AR 72944
479-928-4404

***NORTH SIDE BEHAVIORAL HEALTH AND
SPECIALITY SERVICES**
3202 N. 6th St.
Fort Smith AR 72904
479-783-3900

Website: www.rvpcs.org

*RVPCS - NORTHSIDE CLINIC
4900 Kelley Hwy
Fort Smith AR 72904
479-785-5700

Website: www.rvpcs.org

+GOOD SAMARITAN CLINIC
615 North B Street
Fort Smith AR 72901
479-783-0233

SEBASTIAN COUNTY - FORT SMITH WIC CLINIC
6601 Phoenix Ave
Fort Smith AR 72903
479-478-3062

SEBASTIAN COUNTY HEALTH CENTER
3112 S 70th St
Fort Smith AR 72901
479-452-8600

County: Sharp County, AR

CAVE CITY MEDICAL CLINIC
301 S. Main St.
Cave City AR 72521
870-283-5353

HARDY MEDICAL CLINIC
195 Hospital Drive, Ste. A
Cherokee Village AR 72525
870-257-6060

MAINLINE HEALTH SYSTEMS - PORTLAND
HEALTH CENTER
223 N. Main St.
Portland AR 71663
870-737-2221

MIDWAY MEDICAL CLINIC
195 Hospital Drive
Cherokee Village AR 72525
870-257-6000

WRMC MEDICAL COMPLEX
195 Hospital Drive Ste d
Cherokee Village AR 72525
870-257-6030

County: Union County, AR

INTERFAITH CLINIC
403 West Oak Suite 200
El Dorado AR 71730
870-864-8010

*+STRONG CLINIC
253 S Concord St
Strong, AR 71765
Website: cabun.org
Telephone Number: 870-797-7620
Appointment Number: 870-798-4064

County: Van Buren County, AR

*+BMRHC - CLINTON CLINIC
465 Medical Center Pkwy
Clinton, AR 72031
Website: www.bmrhc.org
Telephone Number: 501-745-7888
Appointment Number: 870-448-3796

*+BOSTON MOUNTAIN RURAL HEALTH CTR
110 Village Ln
Fairfield Bay, AR 72088
Website: www.bmrhc.org
Telephone Number: 501-884-6898
Appointment Number: 870-448-3796

HOPE MEDICAL CLINIC
145 Shake Rag Rd
Clinton AR 72031
501-745-7161

County: Washington County, AR

*+COMMUNITY CLINIC SPRINGDALE DENTAL
610 E Emma Ave
Springdale, AR 72764-4634
Website: www.communityclinicnwa.org

Telephone Number: 479-751-7417
Appointment Number: 479-751-7417 x6069

*+COMMUNITY CLINIC SPRINGDALE
MEDICAL
614 E Emma Ave Ste 300
Springdale, AR 72764-4469
Website: www.communityclinicnwa.org
Telephone Number: 479-751-7417
Appointment Number: 479-751-7417 x6069

+NORTHWEST ARKANSAS FREE HEALTH
CENTER
10 South College Avenue
Fayetteville, AR 72701
Telephone Number: 479-444-7548

+St. FRANCIS HOUSE NWA, INC.
614 E Emma Ave. #300
Springdale, AR 72764
Telephone Number: 479-751-7417

County: White County, AR

*ARCARE - 14
2802 Highway 367 N
Bald Knob, AR 72010-3165
Website: www.arcare.net
Telephone Number: 870-724-6207
Appointment Number: 870-347-2534

*+BALD KNOB MEDICAL CLINIC
170 Highway 167 N
Bald Knob, AR 72010-4058
Website: www.wrrhc-ar.org
Telephone Number: 501-724-6207
Appointment Number: 870-347-2534

KENSETT MEDICAL CLINIC - ARCARE
606 Wilbur D. Mills N.
Kensett AR 72082
Telephone Number: 870-742-5697

*SEARCY FAMILY HEALTH CENTER-
ARCARE
406 Rodgers Dr
Searcy, AR 72143-7433
Website: www.wrrhc-ar.org
Telephone Number: 501-279-7979
Appointment Number: 870-347-2534

*+WHITE RIVER MED SERVICE CLINIC
606 W Wilbur Mills Ave
Kensett, AR 72082-9051
Website: www.wrrhc-ar.org
Telephone Number: 501-742-5697
Appointment Number: 870-347-2534

County: Woodruff County, AR

*+AUGUSTA DENTAL CLINIC
623 N 9th St
Augusta, AR 72006-2129
Website: www.wrrhc-ar.org
Telephone Number: 870-347-25 08
Appointment Number: 870-347-2534

*+COTTON PLANT MEDICAL CLINIC-
ARCARE
125 Oak St
Cotton Plant, AR 72036
Website: www.wrrhc-ar.org
Telephone Number: 870-459-3588
Appointment Number: 870-347-2534

*MCCRORY HEALTH CENTER- ARCARE
801 N Edmonds
McCrory, AR 72101
Website: www.wrrhc-ar.org
Telephone Number: 870-731-5411
Appointment Number: 870-347-2534

*+WHITE RIVER RURAL HEALTH CENTER, INC.
623 N 9th St
Augusta, AR 72006-2129
Website: www.wrrhc-ar.org
Telephone Number: 870-347-2534
Appointment Number: 870-347-2508

*WHITE RIVER RURAL HEALTH WELLNESS
904 N 4th St
Augusta, AR 72006-2039
Website: www.wrrhc-ar.org
Telephone Number: 870-347-1137
Appointment Number: 870-347-2534

County: Yell County, AR

RIVER VALLEY CHRISTIAN CLINIC
1714 St Hiwy 22 W
Dardanelle AR 72834
479-229-2566

DISCLAIMER

This Book is Not Legal Advice. This information is general in nature and should not be relied on as a substitute for legal advice. This book is provided as an education service by Law Offices of Lisa Douglas.

These clinics are in no way affiliated with Law Offices of Lisa Douglas, Inc. These clinics may have changed their status since the printing of this book. It is recommended you call these clinics in advance to determine their status before relying upon this book.

www.ingramcontent.com/pod-product-compliance
Lightning Source LLC
Chambersburg PA
CBHW070822290526
45795CB00002B/806